THE ANAL MANUAL

Step by step guide to enjoying and exploring anal sex

LOUISE EVANS

TABLE OF CONTENT

CHAPTER ONE

INTRODUCTION TO ANAL SEX

Anal sex is a form of sexual activity in which the penis is inserted into the anus.It can be a pleasurable experience for both partners, although it is important to take the necessary steps to ensure the experience is safe and enjoyable. In this guide, we'll discuss how to prepare for anal sex, the potential risks involved, and how to make it an enjoyable experience. We'll also provide some tips for couples who are interested in exploring anal sex.

DEFINITION

Anal sex is the term used to describe sexual penetration of the anus. It is a form of sexual activity that can be enjoyed by both heterosexual and homosexual couples. Anal sex can be pleasurable for both partners when it is done correctly. For people who are new to anal sex, it is important to take things slow and use plenty of lubrication.

BENEFITS OF ANAL SEX

1. Increased pleasure: For both partners, anal sex can provide a unique sensation due to the placement of nerve endings in the anus and rectum. This can enhance the pleasure experienced during sexual activity. Because there are a lot of nerve endings in the anus that can give you a different feeling, it can be enjoyable

2. Improved intimacy: Anal sex can be an intimate experience for partners due to the close physical contact and increased communication that is often necessary to make the experience enjoyable

3. Increased stimulation: Anal sex can provide increased stimulation due to the unique feeling of tightness that can be experienced.

4. Enhanced orgasmic pleasure: Anal sex can provide a different kind of orgasmic pleasure for both men and women due to the placement of nerve endings in the rectum.

5. Increased trust: Anal sex can increase trust between partners due to the vulnerability of the experience and the communication required to make it enjoyable.

RISKS OF ANAL SEX

When engaging in anal sex, it is also essential to use a condom or another barrier method to help lower the risk of sexually transmitted infections (STIs) and other infections.

1. Increased risk of spreading sexually transmitted infections (STIs): Anal sex can put both partners at risk for infections and sexually transmitted diseases (STIs). Anal sex carries the highest risk of transmitting STIs such as HIV, gonorrhea, chlamydia, and herpes, due to the fragile skin in the anus and rectum.

2. Damage to the rectum: The rectum is not meant to accommodate a penis, and its walls are much more fragile than those of the vagina. Unprotected anal sex can cause pain, tearing, and bleeding if done incorrectly or too quickly due to the sensitivity of the anus and rectum.

3. Unwanted pregnancy: Anal sex does not provide protection against pregnancy. If semen enters the vagina during anal sex, it can lead to pregnancy.

4. Risk of fecal incontinence: Anal sex can weaken the muscles around the anus, leading to fecal incontinence. This can cause accidental leakage of feces and can be embarrassing and uncomfortable.

SAFETY AND HEALTH

Anal sex is generally considered a safe sexual practice when practiced properly. However, there are some risks associated with anal sex, such as the risk of infection, tearing of the anal tissue, and transmission of sexually transmitted infections (STIs).

It is important to use a water-based lubricant to reduce friction, which can increase the risk of tearing the delicate anal tissue. Also, condoms should be used for any penetrative sex to reduce the risk of STIs.

It is also important to go slowly to reduce the risk of tearing the anal tissue. It is also a good idea to take breaks during anal sex to allow the body to adjust and relax.

Finally, it is important to be aware of the signs of infection and to seek medical attention if any symptoms occur. Symptoms of infections may include pain, itching, discharge, and bleeding.

PREPARATION FOR ANAL SEX

MENTAL PREPARATION

1. Talk with your partner about your mutual expectations and boundaries before engaging in any sexual activity.

2. Take your time and focus on relaxation. Engaging in foreplay and using lubricant can help.

3. Begin with gentle touches and slow, shallow movements. This can help you get used to the sensation and help you relax.

4. Stimulate the area around the anus with your fingers or a sex toy before attempting penetration.

5. Breathe deeply and focus on the sensations you are feeling. If anything becomes too uncomfortable or painful, stop.

6. Communicate with your partner and check in regularly to ensure that everyone is comfortable and enjoying themselves.

PHYSICAL PREPARATION

1. Create a safe and comfortable environment: Make sure to create an environment that is both physically and emotionally safe for both partners. This means putting away any distractions and setting the mood by dimming the lights, playing some music, and using lubricants and condoms.

2. Practice good hygiene: Make sure to practice good hygiene before engaging in any sexual activity. This includes washing the genitals, anus, and surrounding areas with warm water and soap.

 3. Use lubrication: Lubrication is essential for anal sex as the anus does not naturally lubricate itself like the vagina does. Make sure to use a water-based lubricant to reduce friction and make the experience more pleasurable.

4. Communicate: Communication is key for any sexual activity. Make sure both partners are comfortable and consenting before engaging in any activity.

5. Start slow: Start off slow and gentle. It is important to start with external stimulation and to give the anus time to adjust and relax before attempting penetration

 6. Relax: Relaxation is key when it comes to anal sex. Make sure to breathe deeply and concentrate on relaxing the muscles of the anus and lower back to make penetration easier.

7. Use a condom

CHAPTER TWO

ANAL SEX POSITIONS

The Doggy Style - The classic anal sex position, doggy style is all about the pleasure of the receiving partner. The partner on the receiving end gets on all fours while the penetrating partner enters from behind

Doggy style anal sex is a popular sexual position in which the receiving partner is on all fours, facing away from the penetrating partner. It is a very intimate position that allows for deep penetration and clitoral stimulation. This position can be very enjoyable for both partners, as the receiving partner can control the depth and speed of penetration. The penetrating partner also has a great view of the receiving partner's buttocks and can use their hands to stimulate the area.Doggy style anal sex can be quite intense and should be done with caution. It is important to use plenty of lube to reduce any discomfort and to always practice safe sex. It is also important to communicate with your partner during the act to ensure that both parties are comfortable.

Spooning - This intimate position requires the partners to lie side-by-side, with the penetrating partner entering from behind. This position allows the receiver to be in control of the speed and depth of penetration.

Spooning is a great way to enjoy anal sex! This position allows for deep penetration, and is great for those who are looking for a slower, more intimate experience. To get into the spooning position, the receiving partner should lay on their side with the penetrating partner behind them. The penetrating partner can then enter the receiving partner from behind, and the two can move together in a rocking motion. This position can be great for G-spot stimulation, and allows the partners to control the depth and speed of penetration. Spooning can also be a great position for anal play, as the receiving partner can be in control of how much of the penetration they can handle. With the right amount of communication and patience, this can be a great way to enjoy anal sex!

Sitting - This position requires the penetrating partner to sit with their legs outstretched and the receiving partner to straddle them. This allows the receiving partner to control the speed and depth of penetration

In the sitting anal sex position, the receiving partner sits on their partner's lap with their back facing them. The partner can then enter the receiving partner from behind. Both partners can use their hands to stimulate the other partner's erogenous zones. This position can be used to explore anal play and to vary the angles of penetration.

Reverse Cowgirl - In this twist on cowgirl, the receiving partner is on top but facing away from the penetrating partner. This allows the receiving partner to control the speed and depth of penetration.

The penetrating partner is on their back while the receiving partner straddles them and faces away. This position allows the receiver to control the depth and angle of penetration, making it a great choice for those who enjoy anal sex. It is important to use plenty of lubrication and to proceed slowly in order to avoid any discomfort.

Anal Missionary - This position requires the receiving partner to lie on their back with their legs in the air. The penetrating partner then enters from a kneeling position. This position allows for deeper penetration and can be very int**imate.**

Anal missionary sex position is a variation of the traditional missionary position. It involves the receiving partner lying on their back with the penetrating partner on top, but instead of the penetrating partner entering the receiving partner's vagina, they enter their anus.

This position is great for those who enjoy anal sex and want to explore it further. It allows the penetrating partner to control the depth and angle of penetration, while the receiving partner can use their hands to help guide the motion.

Anal missionary sex can be a great way to experience deeper, more intimate connection between partners. This position also allows for more direct stimulation of the clitoris and G-spot, as well as the opportunity for both partners to watch as the anal penetration occurs.

When engaging in anal missionary sex, it is important for both partners to use a water-based lubricant to reduce friction and increase comfort. It is also important for both partners to communicate about their wants and needs, as well as their boundaries, to ensure the experience is enjoyable for both.

CHAPTER THREE

TIPS AND TECHNIQUES

☐ USING TOYS

1. Start Slow: Start slowly and use plenty of lube. Use smaller toys and gradually increase size.

2. Go for Quality: Invest in toys specifically designed for anal play. Avoid using toys that are not specifically designed for anal use as they may cause injury.

3. Lube Up: Use plenty of lube to ensure a comfortable experience. Water-based lube is the best option for anal play.

4. Communication is Key: Talk to your partner throughout the experience to ensure that you are both comfortable and enjoying the experience.

5. Cleanliness is a Must: Always clean your toys before and after use with warm water and a mild soap.

6. Stimulate the Area: Stimulate the area around the anus before penetration to help relax the sphincter muscles.

7. Know Your Limits: Listen to your body and stop if you experience any pain or discomfort.

8. Take it Slow: Take your time and allow your body to adjust to the feeling of having the toy inside.

9. Experiment and Have Fun: There are many different types of toys to try, so don't be afraid to experiment and have fun.

☐ ANAL MASSAGE

Anal massage is a type of massage that focuses on the anus to provide a pleasurable and relaxing experience. It is often used to relax the muscles of the anus and to increase sensitivity in the area. The massage can also be used to explore and open up the area to new sensations. Anal massage can be a great way to explore the body and increase pleasure. It can also be beneficial for those with anal tension and discomfort, as it can help to release any built up tension in the area.

☐ DIFFERENT TYPES OF STIMULATIONS

1. Manual Stimulation: This type of stimulation involves using your hands or fingers to stimulate the anus, either by rubbing, tapping, or pushing the area.

Manual stimulation is a sexual activity that involves stimulating the anus with the fingers or hands. It can be done by one's self or by one's and partner. Manual stimulation can be a great way to explore the pleasure of anal sex and can include activities such as fingering, rimming, and prostate massage.

When engaging in manual stimulation, it's important to use lube and to go slow. The anus is not self-lubricating and the skin can be delicate and easily irritated, so lube helps to prevent discomfort and injury. Start by massaging the area around the anus and gradually work your way inside. Use your fingers to explore the shape and size of the opening. When you're ready, introduce one finger to the anus and move it in and out. Increase the pressure applied and intensity as you do desire.

Manual stimulation can be used to stimulate the prostate, which is located at the inner wall of the rectum. If you're exploring prostate massage, use your finger to massage the area in a 'come hither' motion. You can also use a toy specifically designed for prostate stimulation.

It's important to keep communication open and to check in with your partner throughout the experience. Before and during the activity, ensure that your partner is comfortable.

2. Oral Stimulation: This involves using your mouth and tongue to stimulate the anus. This can be done with licking, sucking around the anus and the area around it, or using a sex toy.Oral stimulation can increase arousal, provide pleasure, and make the area more relaxed and ready for anal sex. It also helps to create a strong connection and trust between partners. To ensure safety, it is important to use a dental dam or plastic wrap in order to avoid any direct contact between the mouth and anus.

3. Anal Beads: These are a series of beads that are inserted into the anus and then removed. The feeling of the beads being inserted and removed can be quite pleasurable.

Anal beads are a sex toy consisting of multiple beads strung together on a string or rope. The beads are typically inserted into the anus one by one and then removed at varying speeds depending on the desired sensation. Anal beads can be used both by men and women, but they are most commonly used to stimulate the male prostate. Anal beads can provide a variety of pleasures, ranging from gentle massage and stimulation to intense pleasure.

The beads can create a pleasurable feeling of fullness and pressure, as well as intense orgasms. Anal beads can also be used to increase pleasure during masturbation, foreplay, and other sexual activities.

4. Vibrators: Vibrators are specially designed sex toys that can be used to stimulate the anus. They come in a variety of shapes and sizes and can be used for both clitoral and anal stimulation.

Vibrators are a great way to add extra pleasure and sensation to anal sex. They provide incredible pleasure and sensation. Vibrators can help to relax the sphincter muscles, making anal penetration easier and more comfortable. When used in tandem with a lubricant, they can provide an even more pleasurable experience. Additionally, they can be used to stimulate the prostate, which can lead to intense, full-body orgasms. With the right vibrator, anal sex can become an even more enjoyable experience.

4. Prostate Massagers: These are specifically designed to target the male prostate, which can be an extremely pleasurable experience.

Prostate massagers are a great way to enhance anal sex. They are designed to provide targeted stimulation to the male prostate gland. The prostate is an erogenous zone that can provide intense pleasure when stimulated. Prostate massagers come in a variety of shapes and sizes, allowing for a customizable experience. Many are designed with a curve and a bulbous head for direct and effective stimulation. Some even come with vibration or other special features for added pleasure. Prostate massagers can be used alone or with a partner, making them an ideal addition to any anal sex session.

5. Butt Plugs: Butt plugs are inserted into the anus and left in place during sexual activity. Butt plugs are a great way to explore anal sex and can be used to enhance pleasure and intensify sensations during sex. Butt plugs come in a variety of sizes and shapes to accommodate everyone's pleasure preferences. When used properly, butt plugs can provide a variety of pleasurable sensations, from gentle pressure to intense vibrations. They can also help to relax the anal muscles, making anal sex more comfortable and enjoyable. When used in combination with other toys and techniques, butt plugs can add an exciting new dimension to your sex life.

6. Anal Fisting: Anal fisting is a type of anal stimulation where one or more fingers are inserted into the anus and then manipulated. This is typically done with a partner and should be done with caution.

It is considered a form of BDSM (Bondage, Discipline, Sadism, and Masochism). Anal fisting can be a highly intimate and pleasurable experience, as it can provide a deep and intense sensation. However, it is important to note that it is a risky activity, and should only be done with caution and after thorough preparation and communication between partners. It is also important to use a high-quality lubricant, such as silicone-based lube, to reduce the risk of tearing or other damage to the rectal area.

CHAPTER FOUR

TROUBLE SHOOTING

☐ PAIN

Anal sex can cause pain if the receiver is not properly relaxed, if too much force is used, or if the wrong type of lubricant is used. Additionally, if the receiver is not aroused or lubricated enough,
the act can cause tearing and burning sensations. To ensure a comfortable and enjoyable

experience, it is important to use a good amount of lubricant and to go slowly, allowing the receiver to get used to the sensation. Communication between partners is also key to ensure that both parties are comfortable and enjoying themselves.

☐ BLEEDING

Anal sex can be a pleasurable experience for some people, however, it can also cause some people to experience bleeding. This is especially true for those who are new to anal sex. Bleeding from the anus can occur due to the thin and delicate tissue in the rectum being stretched or torn during anal sex. This can cause pain and discomfort and can be quite alarming for some people. If you experience bleeding during anal sex, it is important to stop and seek medical attention if necessary. It is also important to practice safe sex and to use plenty of lubricant to reduce the risk of tearing or injury.

☐ ANXIETY

Anal sex can be an incredibly pleasurable experience, and yet it can also be a source of anxiety for many people. This anxiety can stem from a variety of sources, including fear of the unknown, fear of physical pain, and fear of the social stigma surrounding anal sex.

The best way to reduce your anxiety is to be as informed and prepared as possible. Make sure you understand the risks and benefits associated with anal sex and take the appropriate steps to

ensure safe and pleasurable sexual activity. Talk to your partner about what feels good and what doesn't and be sure to use plenty of lubrication to reduce the risk of physical discomfort.

It's also important to recognize that it's normal to feel anxious about anal sex. Allowing yourself to feel your emotions and accept them can help you to reduce your overall anxiety levels. Remember, anal sex should be consensual and pleasurable for both partners, so don't be afraid to take things slow and enjoy the experience.

AFTERCARE

Aftercare for anal sex is important and can help ensure a positive experience for both partners. Here are some tips to help:

1. Clean Up: Be sure to thoroughly clean up after anal sex. This includes washing and rinsing the anus and genitals with warm water and mild soap. Some couples may also choose to use an enema to clean the rectum.

- ☐ Start by thoroughly washing the anus with warm water and a mild soap. Make sure to get in all the crevices and clean off any feces that may be present.

- ☐ Rinse off the area with warm water and then gently pat the area dry with a clean towel.

- ☐ Apply a light coating of lubricant to the anal area to help protect the skin from any further irritation.

- ☐ To help prevent the spread of bacteria, it is important to use a condom during anal sex. After sex, dispose of the condom properly and wash your hands.

☐ Women should urinate after anal sex to help flush out any bacteria that may have been transferred during sex.

☐ If there is any discomfort or pain after anal sex, apply a cold compress to the area or take an over-the-counter anti-inflammatory to help reduce swelling and pain.

☐ Lastly, make sure to communicate with your partner about any issues or concerns you may have. Anal sex should be an enjoyable experience for both partners, so make sure to discuss any issues that arise and how to prevent them in the future.

2. Take a Break: Aftercare for anal sex should include taking a break. This will give both partners time to relax and reflect on their experience.

Anal sex can be a pleasurable experience for both partners, but it's important to take care of your body afterwards. Taking a break after anal sex is an important part of aftercare and can help your body to recover.

A break can be something as simple as taking a few minutes to relax and cuddle. You can also take a long hot shower, or use a bidet to clean up.

Taking a break can also give you a chance to talk about the experience and make sure both partners are feeling happy, safe and satisfied.

3. Hydrate: After anal sex, it's important to drink plenty of fluids to help replenish any lost water.

Hydrating after anal sex is an important part of aftercare. Drinking plenty of fluids can help to replenish lost liquids and help the body recover from any soreness or discomfort that may have been caused by the experience. Staying hydrated will also help to reduce the risk of infection, as it helps to flush out any bacteria that may have been introduced during the act. It is also important to take a warm shower or bath to help soothe any soreness and clean the area thoroughly. Finally, applying a light lubricant such as coconut oil or olive oil to the area can help to keep it hydrated and reduce any itching or burning sensations.

4. Comfort: Aftercare for anal sex should include comforting the recipient of anal sex. This can be done by providing a massage or simply cuddling.

Aftercare for anal sex is important for both partners, especially for the receiver, who may be feeling vulnerable or sore. Comforting the receiver can help them feel safe and relaxed. This can include cuddling, gentle kisses, and positive affirmations. It is also important to provide the receiver with physical

comfort, such as giving them a warm bath, providing a massage, or using lubricant to reduce discomfort. Talking openly about the experience is encouraged, as it can help to reduce any negative feelings. Lastly, it is important to remind the receiver that they are not alone and that their partner is there to support them.

5. Talk: Aftercare for anal sex should include talking about the experience. This can be done in a way that amounts respects and not from a critic or judgmental view.

Talking about anal sex aftercare is an important part of any sexual encounter. It's important to discuss both physical and emotional aftercare to ensure both partners are comfortable and have a rewarding experience.

Physically, it is important to ensure that the anal area has been properly cleaned after sex. This may involve a warm shower or bath and the use of an enema. It is also important to use a condom during anal sex, to reduce the risk of sexually transmitted infections.

Emotionally, it is important to take the time to talk about the experience and discuss any concerns that either partner may have. Aftercare should be a time of open communication and support, so that the experience is positive for both parties.

Finally, it is important to be mindful of any potential physical or emotional issues that may arise after anal sex. If any pain or discomfort arises, or if either partner feels emotionally uncomfortable after the experience, it is important to discuss this with a doctor or a counsellor. Talking about these issues can help resolve any problems that may arise.

6. Safety: Aftercare for anal sex should include making sure that any toys or tools used were cleaned and stored properly. This will help prevent the spread of any potential infections.

Anal sex can be a pleasurable and safe experience when it is done correctly and with proper precautions. Aftercare is an important step to ensure that both partners involved in the activity remain safe and comfortable.

• Take your time: Anal sex should be slow and intentional. Make sure to communicate with your partner and use plenty of lubrication.

• Clean up: Make sure to wash the anal area with warm water and mild soap after anal sex.

• Avoid rough sex: Do not engage in any rough or forceful activities as this could cause pain and damage to the internal and external areas of the anus.

• Check for injuries: Check the area for any cuts or tears that may have occurred during the activity. If any injuries are present, seek medical attention.

• Use condoms: Condoms are important to use during anal sex to help reduce the risk of STDs and other infections.

• Get tested: Make sure to get tested for STDs and other infections regularly.

• Be aware of emotional triggers: Anal sex can provoke strong emotional responses, so it's important to be aware of any potential triggers for both partners.

• Talk about it: Discuss any preferences, boundaries, and feelings

7. Lubricant: Anal sex can be very uncomfortable without the proper amount of lubricant. Make sure to use a water-based lubricant to help reduce any pain.

Lubricant is an essential part of anal sex, and it is important to use it liberally to ensure a comfortable and enjoyable experience. Aftercare for anal sex

should include cleaning the area with warm water and a gentle soap and patting it dry with a clean towel. Additionally, it is important to apply a generous amount of lubricant to the area to ensure that it is properly lubricated for future sessions. This will help to reduce friction and prevent any discomfort when engaging in anal sex. Additionally, it is important to use a water-based lubricant, as oil-based lubricants can damage the delicate tissues of the anus.

8. Relax: Aftercare for anal sex should include taking a few moments to relax and reflect. This will help both partners to process their experience and enjoy the afterglow.

Relaxing and reflecting on the experience can be a great way to ensure that the experience was enjoyable and meaningful for both partners. Taking time to reflect on the experience can help to process the emotions and sensations felt during the experience, as well as any potential issues that may have arisen. Taking time to relax after anal sex can also help to reduce any potential soreness or discomfort that may have resulted from the experience. Relaxing activities such as taking a hot bath, reading a book, or having a massage can all help to create a calming atmosphere and can help to restore the body and mind. Reflecting on the experience can also help to build deeper understanding and connection

between the two partners, and can help to ensure that both partners feel supported and respected.